Remove Your Heart Blocks without Surgery

Vivek Kamath

ISBN-13:978-1530002986

ACKNOWLEDGEMENT

I am grateful to my mother Late Mrs. Vimala Kamath for giving me the birth because of which I am able to attain this great moment of writing a book on "Remove Heart Blocks Without Surgery". My Mother died of Diabetes and Cardiac Aliment way back in November 2006. Today I am able to cure Diabetes, Heart Ailment, blood pressure, Cholesterol and any respiratory diseases thru Reiki healing method and many other diseases without Medicines. It was unfortunate that I do not have my mother with me. I am sure her departed soul will now be able to rest in peace today by seeing the achievement of her beloved son. My mother's love and affection was a key for me to attain this position today and instrumental in shaping up my life and destiny. I am very thankful to my mother for giving me this great opportunity to serve the world.

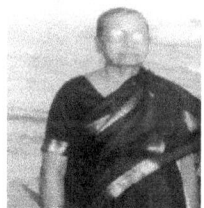

I would like to express my gratitude and heart-full of love to great Reiki Guru and Founder Dr Mikao Usui of Japan.

I would like to thank myself because of my inner strength with which I could able to convert the difficult situations or challenges faced in my life as a great opportunity for learning and always believed that life is a continuous education process. Furthermore, I strongly believed in my life that whatever happens in life it will happen for a good cause and these are based on our good and bad karma/action of past and current life.

Table of Contents

1 Introduction

Background about the Author

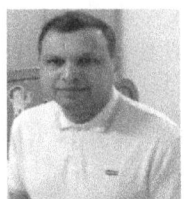

Author Vivek Kamath is an Indian Software Engineer by profession. Author has worked with the world's top International Banks across the globe for nearly 20 years to manage large scale Information Technology (IT) projects. Author is also a Reiki Healing Master Cum Practitioner and Practicing Reiki Healing, Mexican Healing, Crystal Healing, Melchizedek Method of healing from the last 5 years. Author has healed many diabetic patients, blood pressure patients (both high and low blood pressure), Heart Patients (removed the heart blocks), removed kidney stones , cured sinusitis, severe joint pains, constipation, migraines, headaches, insomnia, stomach related problems, diabetic gum problems, skin problems (dry skin, eczema) and chronic nasal allergies, nasal blockages without any medicines. Some of the above treatments have been completed within a week to maximum 1 month duration. Author has intention to help as much as diabetic patients to come out of the disease without any medicines. Author has an intention to build a healing center for diabetic patients across the globe.

For whom was this book prepared?

This book intended for people who are suffering from heart diseases. There are various Healing methods to heal heart diseases.. Author has mentioned about the Reiki Healing in this book.

Author has intention to help as much as patients who are suffering from heart diseases. Author has cured a heart patient who had 3 blocks in his heart. All the 3 blocks have been removed in a span of 21days of healing. In this book, author has given guideline how to heal your heart using Reiki healing method. If in case you are not able to heal by yourself, please feel free to contact author directly by email.

Author has used distant healing method (Patients can reside far away from the healer) of Reiki to heal some of the patients. Distant healing has been found to be very effective.

2 An Overview of our Heart

The heart is the organ that helps supply blood and oxygen to all parts of the body. It is divided by a partition into two halves, and the halves are in turn divided into four chambers. The heart is situated within the chest cavity and surrounded by a fluid filled sac called the pericardium. This muscle produces electrical impulses that cause the heart to contract, pumping blood throughout our body.

What are the role of Blood Vessels?

Blood Vessels are intricate networks of hollow tubes that transport blood throughout our body. The following are some of the blood vessels associated with the heart:

Arteries:

Aorta – is one of the largest artery in our body of which most major arteries branch off from.

Brachiocephalic Artery blood from the aorta to the head, neck and arm regions of the body.

Carotid Arteries - supply oxygenated blood to the head and neck regions of the body.

Common iliac Arteries – This arteries carries oxygenated blood from the abdominal aorta to the legs and feet.

Coronary Arteries – This arteries mainly carries oxygenated and nutrient filled blood to the heart muscle.

Pulmonary Artery – This artery carries de-oxygenated blood from the right ventricle to the lungs.

Subclavian Arteries – This artery is key in terms of supplying oxygenated blood to the arms.

Veins:

Brachiocephalic Veins- is nothing but two large veins that join to form the superior vena cava.

Common iliac Veins - veins that join to form the inferior vena cava.

Pulmonary Vein – This vein transport oxygenated blood from the lungs to the heart.

Venae Cavae – This vein transport de-oxygenated blood from various regions of the body to the heart. Please see the below heart system components diagram in the next page.

What is Cardiac Cycle ?

The cardiac cycle is the sequence of events that occurs when the heart beats. There are two phases of the cardiac cycle. In the diastole phase, the heart ventricles are relaxed and the heart fills with blood. In the systole phase, the ventricles contract and pump blood to the arteries. One cardiac cycle is completed when the heart fills with blood and the blood is pumped out of the heart.

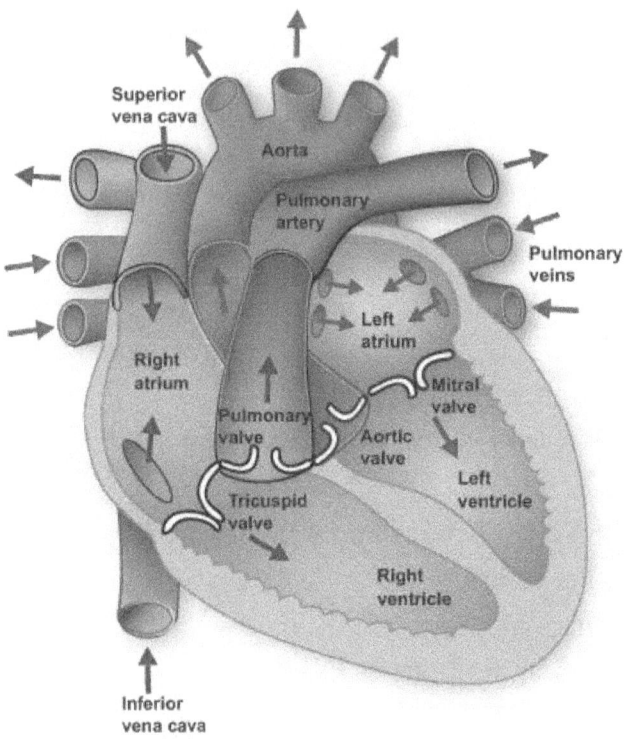

Superior
vena cava

Aorta

Pulmonary
artery

Pulmonary
veins

Right
atrium

Left
atrium

Mitral
valve

Pulmonary
valve

Aortic
valve

Left
ventricle

Tricuspid
valve

Right
ventricle

Inferior
vena cava

Diagram – Heart System Components

What is Cardiovascular System?

The cardiac cycle is key to proper cardiovascular function.
comprised of the heart and the circulatory system, the
cardiovascular system transports nutrients to and removes
gaseous waste from the cells of the body. Our heart and its
cardiac cycle provide the "muscle" needed to pump blood
throughout the body, while blood vessels act as gateways to
transport blood to its destination. The driving fact behind the
cardiac cycle is cardiac conduction. Cardiac conduction is

the electrical system that powers the cardiac cycle and the cardiovascular system.

3. What is heart disease and how many types of heart diseases are there?

Heart disease is a group term for any type of disorder that affects the heart. Heart disease means the same as **cardiac disease** but not **cardiovascular disease**. Cardiovascular disease refers to disorders of the heart and blood vessels while heart disease refers to just the heart.

There are various types of heart diseases. Below are some of the heart diseases.

Angina

Angina (Chest pain) occurs when an area of heart muscle does not get enough oxygen. The patient experiences chest discomfort, tightness or pain. Angina is not technically a disease, but rather a symptom of coronary artery disease. Lack of oxygen to the heart muscle is usually caused by the narrowing of the coronary arteries because of plaque accumulation (atherosclerosis).

Arrhythmia

Arrthythmia is an irregular heartbeat.
Tachycardia is when our heart beats too fast
Bradycardia is when our heart beats too slowly

Premature contraction occurs when the heart beats too early
Fibrillation is occurs when the heart beat is irregular

Arrhythmias are problems with heart-rhythm. They happen when the heart's electrical impulses that coordinate heartbeats do not work as required, making the heart beat in a way it should not, either too fast, slowly or erratically.
Irregular heartbeats are common, we all experience them. They feel like a palpitation.

Congenital heart disease

This is a general term for some birth defects that affect how the heart works. Congenital means we are born with it. Examples include :
Septal defects - there is a hole between the two chambers of the heart. This condition is sometimes called **hole in the heart.**
Obstruction defects - the flow of blood through various chambers of the heart is slightly or even totally blocked
Cyanotic heart disease - not enough oxygen is passed around the body because there is a defect (or some defects) in the heart.

Coronary artery disease

The coronary arteries, which supply the heart with nutrients, oxygen and blood become diseased or damaged, usually because of plaque deposits (Plaque accumulation narrows the coronary arteries and the heart is not able to obtain enough oxygen.

Dilated cardiomyopathy

In this disorder the heart chambers become dilated because the heart muscle has become weak and cannot pump blood properly. The most common reason is not enough oxygen supply reaching the heart muscle (ischemia) due to coronary artery disease. Normally, the left ventricle is affected.

Myocardial infarction

It is also known as heart attack, cardiac arrest *or* infarction and coronary thrombosis. Interrupted blood flow (lack of oxygen) damages or destroys part of the heart muscle. This is usually caused by a blood clot that develops in one of the coronary arteries. Coronary arteries are the blood vessels that passes the heart with the blood.

Heart failure

It is also known as **congestive heart failure**. The heart does not supply blood around the body efficiently. The left or right side of the body might be affected; sometimes both sides are. Coronary artery disease or hypertension (high blood pressure) can over time leave the heart too stiff or weak to fill and supply the blood properly.

Hypertrophic cardiomyopathy

A genetic disorder in which the wall of the left ventricle becomes thick, making it harder for blood to leave the heart. The heart has to work harder to pump blood. This is the leading cause of sudden death in athletes. A father or mother with hypertrophic cardiomyopathy has a 50% chance of passing the disorder onto their children.

Mitral regurgitation

It is also known as **mitral valve regurgitation**, **mitral insufficiency** or **mitral incompetence** occurs when the mitral valve in the heart does not close tightly enough, allowing blood to flow back into the heart. Blood cannot pass through the heart or the body efficiently. Patients may feel very tired and/or not able to breath.

Mitral valve prolapse

The valve between the left atrium and left ventricle does not fully close, it bulges upwards or back into the atrium. Most of the times this condition is not life-threatening and there is no treatment. Some patients, especially if the condition is marked by mitral regurgitation, may require immediate treatment.

Pulmonary stenosis

It is difficult for the heart to pump blood from the right ventricle into the pulmonary article because the pulmonary valve is too tight; the right ventricle has to do more work to overcome the obstruction. A baby with severe stenosis can become cyanotic (turn blue). If pressure in the right ventricle is too high treatment is required. Open Heart Surgery or a Balloon valvuloplasty may be recommended.

4. Symptoms of Heart Diseases

Below are the typical symptoms of heart diseases.

1. Chest pain or angina.
2. Feeling heaviness, pressure and burning sensation in chest.
3. Sweating.
4. Fast and irregular heartbeats.
5. Feeling shortness in breath.
6. Feeling fullness and indigestion.
7. Faint.

Symptoms for Heart Block

Signs and symptoms depend on the type of heart block you have. First-degree heart block may not cause any symptoms. Signs and symptoms of second- and third-degree heart block include:

- Fainting
- Dizziness or light-headedness
- Fatigue (tiredness)
- Shortness of breath
- Chest pain

Symptoms of Coronary Heart Disease(CHD)

Angina - Angina is a chest pain or discomfort that occurs when your heart muscle doesn't get enough oxygen-rich blood

Symptoms of Broken Heart Syndrome

- Chest pain
- Shortness of breath

Symptoms of Arrhythmia

- Too fast heart beat or too slow with an irregular rhythm
- Fluttering or thumping feelings or skipped beats in the chest (called palpitations)
- Suddenly stop beating called sudden cardiac arrest (SCA).

Symptoms of Heart Attack

- Chest pain or discomfort.
- Back or neck pain, indigestion, heartburn, nausea, vomiting, extreme tiredness or breathing problems
- Light-headedness
- Dizziness
- Discomfort in one or both arms, the back, neck, jaw, or upper part of the stomach
- Pain in the left arm and cold sweat

Symptoms of Heart Failure

- Shortness of breath
- Fatigue
- Sweating in the feet, ankles, legs, abdomen and veins in the neck

5. Causes of Heart Diseases

Type of Heart Disease	Causes
Coronary Heart Disease (CHD)	Smoking (both active and passive smoking) High amount of certain fats and cholesterol in the blood High blood pressure Blood vessel inflammation High blood glucose level in the blood
Cardio Vascular Disease	An Unhealthy Diet Lack of exercise Obesity Smoking and Alcohol consumption
Heart arrhythmia	Heart defects - born with (congenital heart defects) Coronary artery disease High blood pressure Diabetes Smoking Excessive use of alcohol or caffeine Drug abuse Stress
Congenital heart defects	Genetic reasons.
Cardiomyopathy	**Dilated cardiomyopathy.** Reduced blood flow to the heart (ischemic heart disease), infections, toxins and certain drugs Genetics **Hypertrophic cardiomyopathy**

	High Blood Pressure
	Ageing
	Restrictive cardiomyopathy
	Connective tissue disorders
	Hemochromatosis
	By some cancer treatment side effects
Heart infection	Bacteria
	Viruses
	Parasites
Valvular heart disease	Rheumatic fever
	Infections (infectious endocarditis)Connective tissue disorders

6. Test for Heart Diseases

1. EKG (Electrocardiogram)

An EKG is a simple test that detects and records the heart's electrical activity. The test shows how fast the heart is beating. An EKG also records the strength and timing of electrical signals as they pass through the heart.

An EKG can show us some signs of heart damage due to Chronic heart disease (CHD) and signs of a previous or current heart attack.

2. Stress Testing/TMT (Thread Mill Test)

A stress test can show possible signs and symptoms of CHD, such as:

- Abnormal changes in your heart rate or blood pressure
- Shortness of breath or chest pain
- Abnormal changes in your heart's function

The report of stress tests shows how well blood is flowing in your heart and how well our heart pumps blood when it beats.

3. Echocardiography

Echocardiography (echo) uses sound waves to create a moving picture of our heart. The test provides information about the size and shape of our heart and how well our heart chambers and valves are working.

Echo also can show areas of poor blood circulation in the heart, areas of heart muscle that aren't contracting normally, and previous injury to the heart muscle caused by poor blood flow.

4. Chest X Ray

A Chest X Ray creates pictures of the organs and structures inside our chest, such as our heart, lungs, and blood vessels. A chest x ray can reveal signs of heart failure, as well as lung disorders. If there are any other CHD it can be tracked with the chest x-ray.

5. Blood Tests

Blood tests check the levels of certain fats, Cholesterol lipids(LDL, HDL,VLDL etc.), sugar, and proteins in our blood. Abnormal levels may be a sign that patients are at risk for CHD.

During a heart attack or failure, heart muscle cells die and release proteins into the bloodstream. Blood tests can measure the amount of these proteins in the bloodstream. High levels of these proteins are a sign of a recent heart attack.

6. Coronary Angiography and Cardiac Catheterization

Coronary Angiography tests or factors suggest whether the patient have CHD. This test uses special x rays to look inside picture of our coronary arteries.

To get the dye/special x-rays into our coronary arteries, GP(General Practitioner) will use a procedure called cardiac catheterization.

A very thin, flexible tube called a catheter is put into a blood vessel in our arm, groin (upper thigh), or neck. The tube is threaded into our coronary arteries, and the dye is released into our bloodstream. Coronary angiography detects blockages in the large coronary arteries.

7. Cardiac MRI stress test (magnetic resonance imaging) stress test.

Cardiac MRI test uses radio waves, magnets, and a computer to create pictures of our heart as it pumps. The test produces both still and moving pictures of our heart and major blood vessels.

7. Complication of Heart Diseases

Heart Failure

Heart failure occurs when the heart cannot adequately pump blood throughout the body. This can cause shortness of breath, dizziness, faintness ,confusion, and the buildup of fluid in the body, causing swelling.

Heart Attack

A heart attack occurs when the coronary arteries narrow so much that they cut off blood supply to the heart. The heart cells begin to die as they are deprived of oxygen. Symptoms include shortness of breath and severe chest pain that may radiate to the back, jaw, neck or left arm.

Stroke

When the heart isn't working effectively, blood clots are more likely to form in the blood vessels. A stroke occurs when one of these clots forms in a blood vessel in the brain and cuts off blood flow.
Below are some of the stroke symptoms include:
- numbness on one side of the body
- confusion
- trouble speaking
- loss of balance or coordination

Pulmonary Embolism

A pulmonary embolism is similar to a stroke, here the blocked blood vessel is in the lungs instead of the brain. Symptoms include shortness of breath, chest pain on breathing, and bluish skin.

Cardiac Arrest

Cardiac arrest occurs when the heart suddenly stops functioning. It's usually caused by an electrical disturbance in the heart. Arrhythmias caused by heart disease can lead to cardiac arrest. This will lead to death if not treated immediately.

Peripheral Artery Disease (PAD)

The same narrowing that occurs in coronary artery disease can happen in the arteries that supply blood to the arms and legs. The main symptom of PAD is severe leg pain while walking.

8. Global Fact Findings – Heart Diseases

According to Research data heart disease is the leading cause of death in the UK, USA, Canada, India, China, Japan and Australia.

An estimated 17.3 million people died globally from Cardio Vascular Disease (CVD); 30% of all deaths.

USA

1. Heart Disease is the number one cause of death in the United States, resulting in over 787,000 deaths in 2011.

2. The number of US adults diagnosed with heart disease stands at 26.6 million (11.3% of adult population).

3. In the United States, someone has a heart attack **every 43 seconds**.

4. 23.5% of all deaths in the USA today are caused by heart disease.

5. About **610,000 people** die of heart disease in the United States every year–that's **1 in every 4 deaths**.

6. Coronary Heart Disease (CHD) is the most common type of heart disease, killing over **370,000 people** annually.

7. Coronary heart disease alone costs the United States **$108.9 billion** each year.

United Kingdom

1. In the UK, every year 160,000 people die from heart and circulatory disease out of which 73,000 die from coronary heart disease (CHD)

2. Every 7 minutes someone in the UK will have a heart attack

3. Every 12 minutes someone in the UK will have a stroke

4. 1.2 million Men and 900,000 women are living with chronic angina (pain in the chest)

5. 1 million men and nearly 500,000 women are living with the after effects of a heart attack
6. One third of people who suffer a fatal heart attack die before they can be taken to hospital
7. Overall CVD is estimated to cost the UK economy around 19 billion

Europe

1. Coronary Heart Disease (CHD) is the single most common cause of the death before the age of 65 accounting 16% of male and 10% female deaths.

Japan

1. Heart disease is the second most prominent cause of mortality in Japan and coronary heart disease (CHD) accounts for approximately half of heart disease– related deaths.
2. The CHD mortality rate in Japan has been one-third of the total death.

China

1. According to official data, in China, about 230 million people have cardiovascular disease

2. One in 5 adults in the China has a cardiovascular disease

India

1. Heart diseases have emerged as the number one killer in both urban and rural areas of the India.
2. According to study, 2.4 Million Indians die due to heart disease every year
3. One fifth of the deaths in India are from coronary heart disease.
4. There are an estimated 45 million patients of coronary artery disease in India.

Australia

1. CVD is the leading cause of death and disability in Australia.

9. Cure for Heart Diseases

There are several methods to cure heart diseases without medicines.

Below are the some of the healing techniques used across the world to cure heart diseases. I am highlighting only Reiki Healing and Relevant Yoga's and Mudra's to heal the heart and circulatory system of our body.

A. Reiki Healing

B. Crystal Healing

C. Pranic Healing

D. Mexican Healing

E. Holographic Healing

F. Yoga and Mudra

Reiki Healing for Heart

A.   Reiki Healing

Reiki is a form of alternative medicine developed in 1922 by Japanese Buddhist Dr. Mikao Usui.

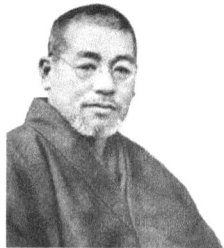

Mikao Usui 臼井甕男(1865–1926)

It uses a technique commonly called palm healing or hands-on-healing.The word Reiki is made of two Japanese words – Rei which means "God's Wisdom or the Higher Power" and Ki which means "life force energy". So Reiki is actually "spiritually guided life force energy or universal energy".

Any heart disease can be completely healed using Reiki Healing. Distant Healing (Patients need not be present in the physical location of the healer/Reiki Practitioner) method found to be very effective. Our heart governs the blood flowing out and in to the heart and body. In terms of Chakra healing, Reiki healer needs to heal the heart chakra of the patient. Also, healer needs to focus on healing the entire heart if there is a significant high blood pressure or even low blood pressure. Healer needs to normalize the systolic and diastolic pressure of the heart. This healing can cure both high blood pressure and low blood pressure. Healer needs to verify the patients report and check the type of disease whether disease is circulatory related or genetic defects etc. If the disease is due to high blood pressure or cholesterol or high diabetes the respective disease and chakra needs to be healed along with healing of heart chakra. Healer also needs to heal the organs specific to this disease. (Apart from the heart, there may be need to heal the kidney, liver, pancreas or lungs.)

With the Reiki, we can set the body clock and timer for removing the negative energies for the life time from the heart's circularly system. By doing this, we can permanently cure any chronic blood related or heart ailments diseases.

Yoga For Blood Pressure

Yoga is a Sanskrit word meaning "union" and is about getting the mind and the body to work together to find balance, harmony and ultimately better health .Yoga is Physical, mental and spiritual practice or discipline which originated in India. Yoga Gurus from India introduced yoga to the western countries.

In 1980's yoga became popular as a system of physical exercise across the western world. Yoga in

Indian Traditions, however is more than physical exercise, it has a meditative and spiritual core.

Yoga can help to calm the mind, which is more important than you probably realize. One of the reason for the heart disease may be a constant source of worry and stress for varying different reasons. Yoga can help you to relax (both mentally and physically) and forget any worries through breathing and meditation.

Yoga moves can specifically help ease heart system related issues. With regular practice, yoga could help to keep your cardiac system working at its best, and prevent any blood related related issues. Please refer to appendix C for the list of yoga's are useful for heart disease.

10. Heart Diseases Healing in Nut-Shell

In Nut-shell Below are the Heart disease healing summary you may need to keep in mind.

Food Diet

1. Follow the Appendix A and B food to eat and not to eat for healthy heart

2. Always make a habit of drinking 3 Liters of water on daily basis. This will help to release the toxic or negative energies from our body.

3. Reduce your salt in-take in diet, increase potassium in-take in diet (provided you do not have other diseases like Kidney diseases). This will control your blood pressure and hence it also takes care of your heart health in long run.

4. Reduce Smoking and In-take of Alcohol

Exercise

1. Conduct those Yoga which helps the Cardiac System healing (provided in book please refer to appendix)
2. Ensure you walk every day for 30 to 45 minutes.

Life Style Changes

1. Practice Yoga or Meditation to reduce your stress, depression and anxiety levels

2. Practice some stress management techniques to reduce stress level

3. If you have time, practice 7 Chakra Meditation weekly once

4. Practice Heart Healing Mudra for 15 minutes daily or thrice a week

5. Practice some deep breathing exercises helps to ease the body circulatory and cardiac systems

6. Practice Reiki Healing on weekly basis helps you to balance all 7 Chakras which keeps you in good mental and physical health

7. Heal your Heart Chakra on regular basis to heal the Cardiac System. If you follow this on regular basis, you will not have any heart problem or blocks . This healing should take care of your any problem related to heart or lungs.

Appendix A Food to be taken for healthy heart governance

	Food	Description
1	Salmon	Salmon, tuna, sardines and mackerel are the heart-healthy foods because they protects against the plaque build-up in the arteries. These fish contain large amounts of omega-3 fatty acids which lower the risk of arrhythmia (irregular heart beat) and arthrosclerosis (plaque build-up in the arteries) and decrease triglycerides and cholesterol.
2	Oatmeal	Oatmeal is high in soluble fiber which can lower cholesterol.
3	Blueberries	Blueberries, strawberries and other berries have compounds known as anthocyanins, flavonoids (which are antioxidants) that has found effective in decreasing blood pressure and dilate blood vessels.
4	Dark chocolate	Dark chocolate contains flavonoids called polyphenols, which may help blood pressure, clotting and inflammation.
5	Citrus fruits	Citrus fruits are also high in vitamin C, which has been linked with a lower risk of heart disease.
6	Soy	Soy products such as tofu and soy milk are a good way to add protein to your diet without unhealthy fats and

cholesterol. Soy products contain high levels of polyunsaturated fats (good for heart health, fiber, vitamins, and minerals. Soy is useful in reducing blood pressure and LDL (Bad cholesterol) in our blood thereby reduces heart diseases.

7	Potatoes	Potatoes are rich in potassium and fiber, which can help lower blood pressure. and risk for heart disease.
8	Tomatoes	Tomatoes are high in heart-healthy potassium. They're a good source of the antioxidant lycopene. Lycopene is carotenoids that may help get rid of "bad" cholesterol, keep blood vessels open, and lower the risk of heart attack.
9	Nuts	This includes almonds, walnuts, pistachios and macadamia nuts all of which contain good fiber. They also contain vitamin E, which helps lower bad cholesterol. Walnuts has omega-3 fatty acids which is very beneficial to have healthy heart.
10	Legumes	Legumes such as beans, lentils, and peas are an excellent source of protein. Legumes also help to control blood sugar level in people with diabetes.
11	Extra-virgin olive oil	Olive oil is a good source of monounsaturated fats, rich in antioxidants and potassium which can help reduce both cholesterol blood sugar levels and heart disease. Olives are

another source of "good" fat.

12	Red Wine	Red wine, is very beneficial to lower heart disease risk. As per research, polyphenol found in red wine, resveratrol, gives that beverage an added benefit.
13	Green Tea	Recent study found that people who drank four or more cups of green tea daily had a 25% reduced risk of cardiovascular disease and stroke compared with people who "seldom" imbibed the beverage.
14	Pears & Apples	Pears are a good source of vitamin C and are rich in fiber.
	Broccoli, spinach and kale	These vegetables are high in carotenoids, which act as antioxidants and free your body of potentially harmful compounds. They're also high in fiber. and contain tons of vitamins and minerals. Kale has some omega-3 fatty acids.
	Flax seeds	Flax seeds are high in omega-3 fatty acids which is good for heart.
	Avocado	This fruit has healthy fat and like olive oil, they're rich in the monounsaturated fats that may lower heart disease risk factors, such as cholesterol.
	Pomegranate	Pomegranate contains numerous antioxidants, including heart-promoting polyphenols and anthocyanins which

Appendix B Food to be avoided for healthy heart governance

Type of Food

1	Deep Fried Foods
2	Micro wave Food
3	Shell Fish, Crab, Lobster and Tiger Prawns
4	Red Meat
5	Cheese, Diary Items and high fat milk
6	Ice Creams
7	Fast Foods
8	Energy Drinks (sweetened fruit drinks, soda, and sports drinks)
9	White Rice, Breads, pastries, pasta made of white flour
10	Canned Food
11	Processed Food

may help stave off hardening of the arteries.

Appendix D Mudra Heart Diseases

Please note the below mudra's for heart diseases.

Method of Apan Vayu Mudra
The tip of the middle finger and ring finger touches the tip of the thumb, while the index finger touches the base of thumb and the little finger stretched out.

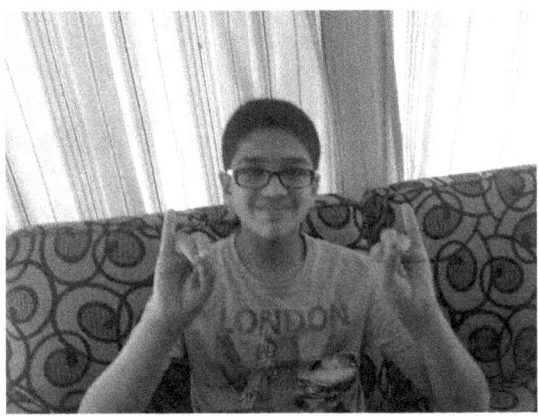

Time Duration:
Practice this mudra daily as many times as you can. Heart patients and blood pressure patients can practice the mudra at least 4 times a day for 15 minutes to see best results.

Benefits
1. It relieves angina/chest pain immediately.
2. It normalizes blood pressure and thus helps in both high and low blood pressure, as it stimulates our circulatory system.
3. In case of palpitations or weak pulse, this mudra will normalize the pulse rate. .
4. It reduces nervousness, as it calms the nervous system.

Appendix C Pranayama & Yoga for heart diseases

I have not documented how to perform these yoga steps in this book. I would advise readers to check with your professional yoga teacher and perform these yoga asana's/poses and pranayama's under their guidance.

There are seven pranayama for heart patients. Pranayama is nothing but a breathing techniques which will cleans our whole body, lungs and heart.

> 1. Bhastrika Pranayama
> 2. Kapalbhati Pranayama
> 3. Bahya Pranayama
> 4. Anulom Vilom Pranayama and Nadi Shodhan
> 5. Udggeth Pranayama
> 6. Pranav Pranayama
> 7. Bhramari Pranayama

Benefits of Pranayama
1. Remove the negative energy, toxins from our body and gives positive energy.
2. Pranayama improves the blood circulation, which is very important for the heart to pump properly.
3. Pranayama calms the mind
4. Cures anxiety and depression
5. Pranayama releases stress and depression
6. Remove artery blockages

Yoga for Heart Patients

1. Uttanapadasana
2. Pavanamuktasana
3. Shavasana

www.ingramcontent.com/pod-product-compliance
Lightning Source LLC
Chambersburg PA
CBHW072024280526
45788CB00007B/2664